NAIL CARE ESSENTIALS

Your Complete Guide to Healthy, Beautiful Nails.

Janaine Lee

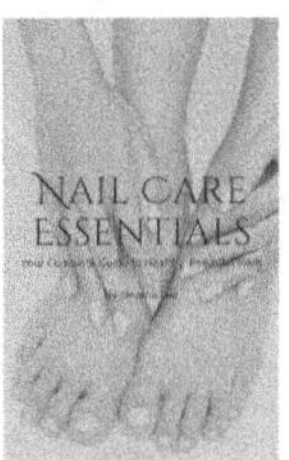

CONTENTS

Introduction

Welcome to "Nail Care Essentials," your comprehensive guide to achieving and maintaining healthy, beautiful nails. This eBook is designed to provide you with the knowledge and tools needed to properly care for your nails, ensuring they remain strong and attractive throughout your life. Whether you're a seasoned nail care enthusiast or just starting on your journey, this guide has something for everyone.

The condition of our nails often reflects our overall health and well-being. Beautiful, well-maintained nails can boost our self-confidence and make us feel more polished and put together. On the other hand, unhealthy nails can make us self-conscious and may even be an indication of underlying health issues. This guide will help you understand the fundamentals of nail care and teach you how to develop a routine that works best for you.

In "Nail Care Essentials," we will cover a wide range of topics, including:

Nail Anatomy and Physiology: Understanding the structure and function of your nails will provide you with a solid foundation for proper care and maintenance. In this section, we'll explore the basic anatomy of your nails, their growth process, and the factors that can influence their health.

Identifying Nail Problems: Recognizing the early signs of nail issues is crucial in addressing them effectively. We'll discuss common nail conditions and disorders, along with their causes, symptoms, and available treatments.

Basic Nail Care Routine: Establishing a consistent nail care routine is the key to achieving strong, healthy nails. This section will guide you through the essential steps of nail care, including trimming, filing, moisturizing, and protecting your nails from damage.

Nail Care Tools and Products: Choosing the right tools and products for your nail care routine can make all the difference. We'll provide an overview of the most important nail care tools, as well as recommendations for the best products to use.

Tips for Strong and Healthy Nails: Learn the secrets to achieving and maintaining strong, healthy nails through proper nutrition, supplements, and lifestyle choices.

Nail Care for Specific Nail Types: Everyone's nails are unique, and what works for one person may not work for another. In this section, we'll discuss specific nail care considerations for different nail types, including brittle nails, thick nails, and nail biters.

Nail Art and Nail Care: Can you have stunning nail art without sacrificing the health of your nails? Absolutely! We'll explore various nail art techniques and provide tips for keeping your nails healthy while expressing your creativity.

By the end of this eBook, you'll have gained a wealth of knowledge on nail care essentials and be well-equipped to take your nail care routine to the next level. So, let's dive in and start your journey towards beautiful, healthy nails!

CHAPTER 1:

NAIL ANATOMY AND HEALTH

1.1 Nail Anatomy

To properly care for your nails, it's essential to understand their structure and how they grow. Nails are made up of a protein called keratin, which is also found in our hair and skin. There are several parts to a nail, including:

Nail plate: The hard, visible part of the nail that is made up of layers of keratin. ("Nail Pitting: What's Going On With Your Fingernails? - Verywell Health") The nail plate is translucent, allowing the underlying nail bed to give it its pinkish color.

Nail bed: The layer of skin beneath the nail plate. It contains blood vessels and nerves, supplying nutrients and oxygen to the growing nail.

Nail matrix: Located beneath the cuticle and at the base of the nail, the matrix is where new nail cells are produced. The health and growth rate of your nails depend on the matrix's health.

Cuticle: A thin layer of dead skin cells that forms a protective barrier between the nail plate and the surrounding skin. The cuticle helps prevent bacteria and fungi from entering the nail matrix.

Lunula: The small, white, crescent-shaped area at the base of the nail. It's the visible part of the nail matrix and indicates the healthy growth of a nail.

1.2 Nail Growth and Factors Affecting It

Nails grow continuously throughout our lives, with fingernails growing faster than toenails. On average, fingernails grow about 3 mm per month, while toenails grow about 1 mm per month. Various factors can influence the growth and health of your nails, including:

Age: Nail growth tends to slow down as we get older.

Diet and nutrition: A balanced diet rich in vitamins and minerals is essential for healthy nail growth.

Health conditions: Certain health issues, such as anemia or thyroid disorders, can impact nail growth and strength.

Medications: Some medications may affect nail health, causing changes in growth rate, texture, or color.

Genetics: Some people naturally have stronger or weaker nails due to their genetic makeup.

Environmental factors: Exposure to harsh chemicals, excessive moisture, or trauma can damage nails and hinder their growth.

1.3 Nail Health Indicators

The appearance of your nails can provide valuable insights into your overall health. Some common nail health indicators include:

Healthy nails: Smooth, pink, and uniform in color, with a slight curve and a smooth, rounded tip.

Brittle or weak nails: Nails that are prone to breaking, peeling, or splitting may indicate a lack of moisture, essential nutrients, or an underlying health issue.

Yellow nails: Discoloration may result from using certain nail products, smoking, or an underlying medical condition.

White spots: These small spots are usually harmless and may be caused by a minor injury to the nail matrix.

Dark lines or spots: If you notice dark lines or spots under your nails that don't grow out, consult a healthcare professional, as they may be a sign of a more serious issue.

In this chapter, we've provided an overview of nail anatomy and the factors that affect nail health. Understanding these basics is crucial for developing a nail care routine that supports healthy growth and prevents damage. In the next chapter, we will delve deeper into identifying common nail problems and how to address them effectively.

CHAPTER 2 :

ADDRESSING NAIL PROBLEMS, PROMOTING HEALTHY NAILS, AND THE IMPACT OF DIET AND NUTRITION

2.1 Common Nail Problems and Conditions

In this section, we will discuss some of the most common nail problems and conditions that may affect your nail health:

Brittle nails: Nails that are prone to breaking, peeling, or splitting can result from a lack of moisture, essential nutrients, or an underlying health issue. To combat brittle nails, keep your nails moisturized and avoid using harsh chemicals.

Ingrown nails: This painful condition occurs when the edge of a nail grows into the surrounding skin, causing inflammation and possible infection. To prevent ingrown nails, trim your nails straight across and avoid cutting them too short.

Fungal infections: Fungi can cause nail infections, leading to discoloration, thickening, and sometimes a foul odor. To prevent fungal infections, keep your nails clean and dry, and avoid sharing nail care tools.

Nail ridges: Vertical or horizontal ridges on your nails may be a result of aging, trauma, or an underlying health issue. Buffing your nails gently can help reduce the appearance of ridges.

Nail psoriasis: This condition presents as pitting, thickening, or discoloration of the nails and is caused by the same factors as skin psoriasis. Treatment may involve topical medications or, in severe cases, systemic medications.

If you notice persistent changes in your nails or experience pain, consult a healthcare professional for a proper diagnosis and treatment plan.

2.2 Maintaining Healthy Nails

To maintain healthy nails, follow these tips:

Keep your nails clean and dry to prevent the growth of bacteria and fungi. ("What Is Breathable Nail Polish and Should You Use It? - L'Oréal Paris")

"Trim your nails regularly and file them in one direction to prevent splitting."(1)

"Moisturize your nails and cuticles with a nourishing oil or lotion."(2)

"Avoid biting your nails or picking at your cuticles, as this can cause damage and infections."(3)

Wear gloves when working with harsh chemicals or water to protect your nails.

Limit the use of nail polish removers containing acetone, as they can cause dryness and brittleness.

Give your nails a break from nail polish occasionally to allow them to breathe and recover.

2.3 Diet and Nutrition for Nail Health

A balanced diet plays a crucial role in promoting healthy nail growth. Consider incorporating these nutrients into your diet for optimal nail health:

Protein: As nails are primarily composed of keratin, a protein, a diet rich in protein can support healthy nail growth. Good sources include lean meats, fish, eggs, dairy products, legumes, and nuts.

Biotin: Biotin, a B-vitamin, has been shown to strengthen nails and promote growth. Foods rich in biotin include eggs, almonds, cauliflower, and whole grains.

Zinc: A zinc deficiency can lead to nail problems such as ridges and white spots. Incorporate zinc-rich foods like oysters, beef, pumpkin seeds, and lentils into your diet.

Iron: An iron deficiency can cause pale or concave nails. Boost your iron intake with foods like red meat, spinach, beans, and fortified cereals.

Vitamin C: This essential nutrient helps with collagen production, which is crucial for nail strength. Citrus fruits, strawberries, bell peppers, and kiwi are all excellent sources of vitamin C.

Omega-3 fatty acids: These healthy fats help keep nails moisturized and flexible. Fatty fish like salmon, mackerel, and sardines, as well as flaxseeds and walnuts, are rich in omega-3s.

In this chapter, we've discussed common nail problems and conditions, tips for maintaining healthy nails, and the role of diet and nutrition in nail health. By following these guidelines, you can promote strong, healthy nails and prevent potential issues.

In addition to a balanced diet, staying hydrated is essential for nail health, as it helps maintain moisture levels in your nails and cuticles. Aim to drink at least eight glasses of water per day to keep your body and nails well-hydrated.

Supplements can also be beneficial for nail health, especially if you have specific nutritional deficiencies. However, it's crucial to consult a healthcare professional before starting any supplementation to ensure it's appropriate for your individual needs.

In the next chapter, we will focus on building a basic nail care routine, including essential steps and best practices for trimming, filing, moisturizing, and protecting your nails from damage. By incorporating these habits into your daily life, you'll be well on your way to achieving beautiful, healthy nails.

CHAPTER 3:

BUILDING A BASIC NAIL
CARE ROUTINE

In this chapter, we will guide you through the essential steps of a basic nail care routine, providing tips and best practices to keep your nails healthy and strong.

3.1 Trimming and Shaping Your Nails

Regular trimming and shaping are crucial for maintaining healthy nails. Follow these steps to trim and shape your nails correctly:

Soften your nails: To make trimming easier and prevent breakage, soak your hands in warm water for a few minutes to soften your nails.

Use clean, sharp tools: Invest in a high-quality pair of nail clippers or nail scissors to ensure a clean, even cut. Always clean and disinfect your tools before and after use.

Trim your nails straight across: Avoid cutting your nails too short or into a curved shape, as this can lead to ingrown nails. Instead, trim them straight across, leaving a little bit of white tip.

Shape your nails: Use a fine-grit nail file to shape your nails, gently filing in one direction to prevent splitting. Round or slightly square shapes with rounded edges are generally the most practical and least prone to breakage.

3.2 Moisturizing Your Nails and Cuticles

Moisturizing your nails and cuticles is vital to prevent dryness, brittleness, and cracking. Follow these tips to keep your nails and cuticles hydrated:

Apply a nourishing oil or lotion: Use a cuticle oil, hand cream, or even coconut oil to moisturize your nails and cuticles. Apply the product daily, massaging it gently into your nails and cuticles to promote absorption and blood circulation.

Protect your hands: "Wear gloves when washing dishes, cleaning, or doing any activity that exposes your hands to water or harsh chemicals for extended periods."(4)

Avoid overusing nail polish remover: Nail polish removers, particularly those containing acetone, can dry out your nails and cuticles. Limit your use of nail polish remover and opt for acetone-free alternatives when possible.

3.3 Nail Protection and Maintenance

Protecting your nails from damage and maintaining their health is an essential part of your nail care routine. Here are some tips to help you protect and maintain your nails:

Wear gloves: Use gloves when working with water, chemicals, or during activities that could cause trauma to your nails.

Avoid using your nails as tools: Refrain from using your nails to open packages, scrape off labels, or perform tasks that could cause them to break or chip.

Maintain a balanced diet: As discussed in Chapter 2, a balanced diet rich in essential nutrients is crucial for healthy nail growth.

Stay hydrated: Drink plenty of water to maintain your overall health and support your nails' moisture levels.

Apply a base coat and topcoat: When applying nail polish, use a strengthening base coat to protect your nails and a topcoat to prevent chipping and prolong the polish's longevity.

In this chapter, we've outlined the essential steps for building a basic nail care routine that promotes healthy, strong nails. By incorporating these practices into your daily life, you'll be well on your way to achieving and maintaining beautiful, healthy nails. In the following chapter, we will discuss nail care tools and products that can help you further enhance your nail care routine.

CHAPTER 4:

NAIL CARE TOOLS AND PRODUCTS

Having the right tools and products is essential for an effective nail care routine. In this chapter, we will introduce you to the most important nail care tools and offer recommendations for selecting the best products for your needs.

4.1 Essential Nail Care Tools

Here are the key tools you should have in your nail care toolkit:

Nail clippers or scissors: Invest in a good-quality pair of nail clippers or scissors for clean, precise cuts when trimming your nails.

Nail file: A fine-grit nail file is essential for shaping your nails and smoothing their edges. Look for a file with a grit level between 180 and 240 for the best results.

Cuticle pusher: A cuticle pusher is a small, flat tool used to gently push back your cuticles without causing damage. Opt for a stainless steel or glass cuticle pusher for durability and easy cleaning.

Cuticle nipper: This small, plier-like tool is used to trim excess or overgrown cuticles. Choose a high-quality stainless steel cuticle nipper with a sharp, precise edge.

Buffer: A nail buffer is a rectangular block with different grit levels on each side. It's used to smooth the surface of your nails, remove ridges, and add shine.

Orange stick: This wooden or plastic stick, often with a pointed end and a flat end, can be used for cleaning under your nails or applying nail products.

4.2 Nail Care Products

In addition to the essential tools mentioned above, consider incorporating these nail care products into your routine:

Cuticle oil or cream: Cuticle oils and creams help to moisturize and nourish your cuticles and nails, promoting healthy growth. Look for products containing natural ingredients like jojoba oil, vitamin E, and almond oil.

Hand cream or lotion: A good-quality hand cream or lotion can help keep your hands, nails, and cuticles moisturized. Choose a product that is non-greasy and absorbs quickly for the best results.

Strengthening base coat: A strengthening base coat can protect your nails from staining and damage caused by nail polish. Look for products containing ingredients like biotin or keratin, which can help strengthen your nails.

Topcoat: A topcoat is essential for sealing in your nail polish and prolonging its wear. Opt for a quick-dry or long-lasting topcoat, depending on your needs and preferences.

Nail polish remover: Choose an acetone-free nail polish remover to prevent drying out your nails and cuticles. There are also nourishing removers available, which contain moisturizing ingredients like glycerin or vitamin E.

In this chapter, we've discussed essential nail care tools and products that can help you build and maintain an effective nail care routine. By investing in high-quality tools and selecting the right products for your needs, you'll be well-equipped to take care of your nails and keep them looking their best. In the next chapter, we will explore tips and strategies for maintaining strong and healthy nails, catering to specific nail types, and incorporating nail art into your routine without compromising nail health.

CHAPTER 5:

TAILORING YOUR NAIL CARE ROUTINE AND INCORPORATING NAIL ART

In this chapter, we will discuss how to customize your nail care routine based on your specific nail type and needs. Additionally, we will explore how to incorporate nail art into your routine while preserving your nail health.

5.1 Customizing Your Nail Care Routine

Everyone's nails are different, so it's important to tailor your nail care routine to your specific needs. Here are some suggestions based on common nail types:

Dry, brittle nails: Focus on moisturizing and nourishing your nails and cuticles. Use cuticle oil, hand cream, and gentle nail polish removers. Avoid acetone-based removers, and give your nails a break from nail polish occasionally.

Soft, weak nails: Strengthen your nails with a strengthening base coat and a diet rich in essential nutrients. Avoid using your nails as tools, and be gentle when filing to prevent further damage.

Thick, ridged nails: Regularly buff your nails to minimize ridges and promote a smoother surface. Use a ridge-filling base coat before applying nail polish to create an even finish.

Discolored nails: Give your nails a break from nail polish to allow them to recover. When using polish, always apply a base coat to prevent staining. If discoloration persists, consult a healthcare professional to rule out any underlying issues.

5.2 Incorporating Nail Art Without Compromising Nail Health

Nail art can be a fun way to express your personal style, but it's essential to ensure that it doesn't compromise your nail health. Here are some tips for incorporating nail art safely:

Use non-toxic nail polishes: Choose nail polishes "that are free from harmful chemicals like formaldehyde, toluene, and dibutyl phthalate" (5) (DBP).

Avoid using glue-on accessories: Gluing accessories like rhinestones or charms onto your nails can weaken them and cause damage. Instead, opt for nail stickers or decals that can be easily removed without causing harm.

Limit the use of nail extensions: While nail extensions can create a dramatic effect, they can also weaken your natural nails. If you choose to use extensions, ensure they are applied by a professional and give your nails a break between applications.

Practice proper removal techniques: When removing nail polish or nail art, avoid picking or peeling, as this can damage your nails. Instead, use a gentle, acetone-free nail polish remover, and be patient during the removal process.

Maintain your nail care routine: Continue to care for your nails even when sporting nail art. Keep your nails and cuticles moisturized, and be mindful of any changes in your nail health.

In this chapter, we've discussed how to tailor your nail care routine to your specific needs and incorporate nail art safely. By customizing your routine and taking precautions when experimenting with nail art, you can maintain healthy, beautiful nails that truly reflect your personal style. As you continue to develop your nail care skills, the next chapter will guide you through DIY nail care recipes, including homemade nail strengtheners and treatments, DIY cuticle oils and creams, and natural hand scrubs and moisturizers.

CHAPTER 6:

DIY NAIL CARE RECIPES

In this chapter, we will explore a variety of DIY nail care recipes that can help you create your own homemade treatments for stronger, healthier nails. We will cover homemade nail strengtheners and treatments, DIY cuticle oils and creams, and natural hand scrubs and moisturizers. These cost-effective and natural solutions can be a great addition to your nail care routine.

6.1 Homemade Nail Strengtheners and Treatments

Olive Oil and Lemon Soak:

2 tbsp olive oil

1 tbsp lemon juice

Mix the olive oil and lemon juice in a small bowl. Warm the mixture in the microwave for a few seconds until it's slightly warm. Soak your nails in the mixture for 10-15 minutes, then rinse and pat dry. The olive oil helps to moisturize and nourish the nails, while the lemon juice brightens and strengthens them.

Tea Tree Oil and Vitamin E Treatment:

5 drops tea tree oil

1 tsp vitamin E oil

Combine the tea tree oil and vitamin E oil in a small container. Apply the mixture to your nails and cuticles daily, massaging it in gently. Tea tree oil has antifungal properties, while vitamin E oil nourishes and strengthens the nails.

6.2 DIY Cuticle Oils and Creams

Jojoba and Lavender Cuticle Oil:

1 tbsp jojoba oil

5 drops lavender essential oil

Mix the jojoba oil and lavender essential oil in a small container. Apply the mixture to your cuticles daily, massaging it in gently. Jojoba oil closely resembles "the natural oils produced by the skin, making it an effective moisturizer,"(6) while lavender essential oil provides a soothing scent.

Coconut and Almond Cuticle Cream:

2 tbsp coconut oil

1 tbsp almond oil

1 tsp beeswax pellets

Melt the coconut oil, almond oil, and beeswax pellets in a double boiler, stirring until combined. Remove from heat and let the mixture cool slightly before transferring it to a small container. Apply the cream to your cuticles daily to nourish and moisturize them.

6.3 Natural Hand Scrubs and Moisturizers

Brown Sugar and Honey Hand Scrub:

1/4 cup brown sugar

2 tbsp honey

1 tbsp olive oil

Mix the brown sugar, honey, and olive oil in a small bowl. Gently massage the scrub onto your hands, focusing on the nails and cuticles. Rinse with warm water and pat dry. This scrub helps to exfoliate and moisturize your hands, leaving them soft and smooth.

Shea Butter and Aloe Vera Hand Cream:

1/4 cup shea butter

2 tbsp aloe vera gel

1 tbsp almond oil

Melt the shea butter in a double boiler, then remove from heat and let it cool slightly. Stir in the aloe vera gel and almond oil until combined. Transfer the mixture to a small container and let it set. Apply the cream to your hands and nails daily to moisturize and soothe the skin.

In this chapter, we've provided a range of DIY nail care recipes that can help you create homemade treatments for your nails, cuticles, and hands. These natural, cost-effective solutions can enhance your nail care routine and contribute to stronger, healthier nails. As you continue on your nail care journey, the following chapters will cover professional nail services, nail care for specific situations, debunking common nail care myths, and expert advice and insights to help you achieve and maintain beautiful, healthy nails.

CHAPTER 7:

PROFESSIONAL NAIL SERVICES

In this chapter, we will discuss the various professional nail services available to help you maintain and enhance your nail health and appearance. We will cover the most common types of services, what to expect during each procedure, and how to choose a reputable salon or technician.

7.1 Types of Professional Nail Services

Manicure: A manicure is a professional treatment that focuses on cleaning, shaping, and polishing the nails. It typically includes soaking the hands, removing any existing nail polish, trimming and filing the nails, pushing back and trimming the cuticles, applying a base coat, nail polish, and topcoat, and finishing with a hand massage.

Pedicure: Similar to a manicure, a pedicure focuses on the care and appearance of the toenails and feet. It includes soaking the feet, removing any existing nail polish, trimming and filing the toenails, pushing back and trimming the cuticles, exfoliating the feet, applying a base coat, nail polish, and topcoat, and finishing with a foot massage.

Gel or Shellac polish: Gel or Shellac polish is a type of nail polish that is cured under a UV or LED lamp, resulting in a long-lasting and durable finish. ("What Is The Difference Between Gel And Regular Nail Polish? [Answered]") It can be applied during a manicure or pedicure and typically lasts for two to three weeks without chipping.

Nail extensions and enhancements: Nail extensions and enhancements are used to add length and/or strength to natural nails. They can be made from various materials, such as acrylic, gel, or fiberglass. The extensions are applied by a professional nail technician and can be filled in every two to three weeks as the natural nails grow.

Nail art: Nail art involves creating intricate designs and patterns on the nails using a variety of techniques, such as hand-painting, stamping, or applying decals. This service can be added to a manicure or pedicure for an additional fee.

7.2 Choosing a Reputable Salon or Technician

To ensure a safe and satisfactory experience when visiting a salon for professional nail services, consider the following factors:

Cleanliness: A reputable salon should prioritize cleanliness and hygiene. Look for clean workstations, sterilized tools, and disposable supplies like nail files and buffers.

Licensing and Certification: Make sure the salon and nail technicians hold the required licenses and certifications for the services they offer. These should be displayed prominently in the salon.

Reviews and Recommendations: Check online reviews and ask for personal recommendations from friends or family members who have visited the salon.

Portfolio: A professional nail technician should have a portfolio showcasing their work. This can help you determine if their style and skill level match your preferences.

7.3 Preparing for and Caring for Professional Nail Services

To get the most out of your professional nail services, follow these tips:

Arrive with clean, bare nails: Remove any existing nail polish before your appointment, and make sure your nails are clean and free of any debris.

Communicate your preferences: Clearly communicate your desired nail shape, length, and color to your technician. Don't be afraid to ask questions or request adjustments during the service.

Follow aftercare instructions: Properly care for your nails following your service to prolong the life of your manicure or pedicure. This may include avoiding water for a specified period, applying cuticle oil regularly, and wearing gloves while doing household chores.

In this chapter, we've discussed the various professional nail services available to help you maintain and enhance your nail health and appearance. With this information, you can make informed decisions about the services that best suit your needs and choose a reputable salon or technician. In the following chapters, we will explore nail care for specific situations, debunk common nail care myths, and share expert advice and insights to help you achieve and maintain beautiful, healthy nails.

CHAPTER 8:

NAIL CARE FOR SPECIFIC SITUATIONS

In this chapter, we will discuss how to care for your nails in different situations and life stages. From pregnancy to nail care for men, we will provide tailored advice and guidance to help you maintain healthy nails, no matter your circumstances.

8.1 Nail Care During Pregnancy

Pregnancy can bring about changes in nail growth and strength due to hormonal fluctuations. Here are some tips for maintaining healthy nails during pregnancy:

Keep nails short and well-groomed: Shorter nails are less prone to breakage and splitting. Trim and file your nails regularly to maintain a manageable length.

Moisturize your hands and cuticles: Hormonal changes may cause dryness in your nails and cuticles. Apply a nourishing hand cream and cuticle oil regularly to keep them hydrated and healthy.

Use non-toxic nail products: Opt for nail polishes and treatments that are free from harmful chemicals like formaldehyde, toluene, and dibutyl phthalate (DBP) to minimize any potential risks to your baby.

8.2 Nail Care for Men

While men's nails tend to be stronger than women's, they

still require proper care and attention. Here are some tips for maintaining healthy nails for men:

Trim and file nails regularly: Keep your nails clean and well-groomed by trimming and filing them regularly. A slightly rounded or square shape with rounded edges is ideal for preventing ingrown nails and breakage.

Moisturize your hands and cuticles: Dry, cracked hands and cuticles are not only uncomfortable but can also lead to infection. Apply a hydrating hand cream and cuticle oil to keep your hands healthy and well-maintained.

Maintain a balanced diet: Eating a balanced diet rich in vitamins and minerals, including biotin, zinc, and iron, will support healthy nail growth and strength.

8.3 Nail Care for Aging Nails

As we age, our nails become more brittle and prone to splitting. Here are some tips for caring for aging nails:

Use a gentle nail file: Instead of a metal nail file, use a fine-grit, cushioned file to minimize damage to your nails.

Keep nails moisturized: Apply a cuticle oil or cream regularly to nourish and hydrate your nails and cuticles.

Avoid harsh nail products: Choose gentle, non-acetone nail polish removers and avoid using nail products containing formaldehyde or other harmful chemicals.

In this chapter, we've discussed how to care for your nails in specific situations and life stages. By adapting your nail care routine to your unique needs, you can maintain healthy nails regardless of the circumstances. In the upcoming chapters, we will debunk common nail care myths and provide expert advice and insights to help you achieve and maintain beautiful, healthy nails.

CHAPTER 9:

NAIL CARE MYTHS DEBUNKED

In this chapter, we will debunk some common nail care myths and misconceptions. By separating fact from fiction, you can make more informed decisions about your nail care routine and ensure you're providing the best care for your nails.

9.1 Myth: Cutting Your Cuticles Is Necessary for Healthy Nails

Truth: Cutting your cuticles can lead to infection and damage the nail matrix, potentially impacting nail growth. Instead of cutting your cuticles, gently push them back with a cuticle pusher or orangewood stick after softening them with cuticle oil or cream.

9.2 Myth: White Spots on Nails Indicate a Calcium Deficiency

Truth: "White spots on nails are typically caused by minor trauma or injury to the nail" (7) matrix, not a calcium deficiency. These spots are harmless and will grow out with the nail.

9.3 Myth: Nails Need to Breathe, So You Should Take Breaks from Wearing Nail Polish

Truth: Nails do not have the ability to "breathe, as they receive oxygen and nutrients from the" (8) bloodstream, not from the air. While it's essential to properly care for your nails and avoid harsh chemicals in nail products, there's no need to take breaks from wearing nail polish for the sake of your nail health.

9.4 Myth: Gel Manicures Ruin Your Nails

Truth: Gel manicures themselves do not ruin your nails. However, improper removal of gel polish can cause damage. To avoid damage, have your gel polish professionally removed or follow the correct removal process at home, which typically involves soaking your nails in acetone and gently lifting the polish off.

9.5 Myth: Filing Nails in a Back-and-Forth Motion Is the Best Way to Shape Them

Truth: Filing your nails in a back-and-forth motion can cause splitting and breakage. Instead, file your nails in one direction, starting from the outer edge and moving toward the center.

In this chapter, we have debunked common nail care myths to help you make more informed decisions about your nail care routine. By understanding the truth behind these misconceptions, you can provide the best care for your nails and avoid potential damage. In the following chapters, we will share expert advice and insights to help you achieve and maintain beautiful, healthy nails.

CHAPTER 10:

EXPERT ADVICE AND INSIGHTS

In this chapter, we will share expert advice and insights to help you achieve and maintain beautiful, healthy nails. From proper nail care techniques to the latest nail trends, these tips from industry professionals will guide you on your nail care journey.

10.1 Tips for Strong, Healthy Nails

Keep your nails clean and dry: Regularly clean your nails with a soft nail brush and soap, and make sure to dry them thoroughly to prevent the growth of bacteria and fungi.

Be gentle with your nails: Avoid using your nails as tools, such as for opening cans or scratching off labels, to prevent breakage and damage.

File your nails properly: File your nails in one direction, starting from the outer edge and moving toward the center. Use a fine-grit, cushioned file to minimize damage.

Moisturize your nails and cuticles: Apply a nourishing cuticle oil or cream daily to keep your nails and cuticles hydrated and healthy.

Wear gloves: Protect your nails and hands from harsh chemicals, water, and dirt by wearing gloves while doing household chores or gardening.

10.2 Nail Care Trends and Innovations

Nail strengtheners and treatments: Products like nail strengtheners and treatments can help improve the health and appearance of your nails by providing essential nutrients and protection.

Breathable nail polish: Breathable nail polish allows water and air to pass through, promoting healthier nails. This type of polish is particularly beneficial for those who wear nail polish frequently or have concerns about nail health.

Gel nail polish alternatives: Newer innovations in nail polish, such as hybrid polishes, combine the benefits of gel and regular nail polish, offering long-lasting wear without the need for UV or LED curing.

Nail art tools and techniques: Nail art continues to evolve, with new tools and techniques, such as stamping plates, nail decals, and magnetic polishes, making it easier to create intricate designs at home.

Eco-friendly and non-toxic nail products: The demand for environmentally friendly and non-toxic nail products has led to the development of nail polishes and treatments free from harmful chemicals like formaldehyde, toluene, and dibutyl phthalate (DBP).

In this chapter, we have shared expert advice and insights to help you achieve and maintain beautiful, healthy nails. By implementing these tips and staying informed about the latest nail care trends and innovations, you can confidently care for your nails and express your personal style. In the final chapter, we will provide guidance on troubleshooting common nail care concerns and offer solutions for addressing these issues.

CHAPTER 11:

TROUBLESHOOTING COMMON NAIL CARE CONCERNS

In this final chapter, we will address common nail care concerns and provide solutions to help you overcome these challenges. From brittle nails to discolored nails, these tips will help you troubleshoot issues and maintain healthy, beautiful nails.

11.1 Brittle or Peeling Nails

Cause: Brittle or peeling nails can be caused by several factors, including excessive exposure to water or harsh chemicals, a lack of moisture, or a deficiency in certain vitamins and minerals.

Solution: To combat brittle or peeling nails, follow these tips:

Keep your nails moisturized with a nourishing cuticle oil or cream.

Wear gloves when doing household chores or gardening to protect your nails from water and chemicals.

Maintain a balanced diet rich in vitamins and minerals that support nail health, such as biotin, zinc, and iron.

11.2 Yellow or Discolored Nails

Cause: Yellow or discolored nails can result from various factors, including prolonged use of dark-colored nail polish, smoking, or an underlying medical condition.

Solution: To address yellow or discolored nails, try these remedies:

Use a base coat before applying nail polish to prevent staining. ("Nail Technician Reveals The Best Methods For Maintaining Strong And ...")

Soak your nails in a mixture of lemon juice and warm water to help lighten discoloration.

If discoloration persists or worsens, consult a healthcare professional to rule out any medical concerns.

11.3 Ingrown Nails

Cause: Ingrown nails occur when the "nail grows into the surrounding skin, causing pain, swelling, and sometimes infection" (9). This can result from improper nail trimming, tight footwear, or genetic predisposition.

Solution: To prevent and treat ingrown nails:

Trim your nails straight across, avoiding overly rounded or sharp corners.

Wear comfortable, well-fitting shoes that provide ample room for your toes.

If an ingrown nail becomes painful or infected, consult a healthcare professional or podiatrist for treatment.

In conclusion, maintaining healthy, beautiful nails requires a consistent nail care routine and an understanding of how to address common concerns. By implementing the tips and advice provided in this ebook, you can confidently care for your nails and achieve the results you desire. Whether you're a nail care novice or a seasoned enthusiast, we hope that "Nail Care Essentials" has provided valuable insights and guidance on your journey to strong, healthy, and beautiful nails.

REFERENCES

1. The Nail C-Curve - NailKnowledge. https://nailknowledge.org/nail-knowledge-base/the-nail-c-curve

2. Brittle nails? Check out natural ways to keep it healthy. https://mirchi.in/stories/lifestyle/natural-ways-to-keep-nails-healthy/99122791

3. Nail Technician Reveals The Best Methods For Maintaining Strong And https://femanin.com/2023/03/29/nail-technician-reveals-the-best-methods-for-maintaining-strong-and-healthy-nails

4. Nail Technician Reveals The Best Methods For Maintaining Strong And https://femanin.com/2023/03/29/nail-technician-reveals-the-best-methods-for-maintaining-strong-and-healthy-nails

5. Vegan nail treatments. - FYNails vegan-friendly nail treatment. https://fynails.com/vegan-nail-treatments/

6. 10 Best Herbs for Dry Skin: Natural Remedies to Soothe and Moisturize. https://www.gafferandchild.com/blogs/blog/10-best-herbs-for-dry-skin

7. Experts Explain Why You May Be Getting Black Lines On Your Nails. https://www.msn.com/en-us/health/medical/experts-explain-why-you-may-be-getting-black-lines-on-your-nails/ar-AA19hHRs

8. Acrylic nails VS gel nails - Which is better?– BTArtbox Nails. https://btartboxnails.com/en-za/blogs/manicure-world/acrylic-nails-vs-gel-nails-1

9. Toenail Problems - Balance Health. https://balancehealth.com/services/toenail-problems/foot-and-ankle-associates/